FOOD AND WELLNESS

How to live a Healthier longer life prevent Diseases, aging and Obesity

Patricia Goodson

Table of contents

Chapter 1

Prologue to food and wellness
Food is fundamental — it offers significant supplements for endurance, and helps the bodywork and remain sound. Food is made out of macronutrients including protein, starches, and fat that not just proffer calories to fuel the body and give it energy but assume specific parts in keeping up with wellbeing.

Food Additionally Offers micronutrients (nutrients and minerals) and phytochemicals that don't create calories yet serve a few fundamental capabilities to ensure the body works ideally.

Macronutrients: Protein, Carbohydrate, and Fat
Protein: Found in dairy product, poultry, game and wild meats, fish and sea foods,

eggs, soybeans and different vegetables utilized in conventional Central American food, protein supports the body with amino acids. Amino acids are the structure blocks of proteins that are required for the development, improvement, fix, and support of human tissues. Protein gives design to muscle and bone, recuperates tissues when harmed, and assists resistant cells with combatting aggravation and disease.

Protein definition
Proteins are moderately large atoms comprising fundamental units called amino acids. Proteins involve carbon, hydrogen, oxygen, nitrogen, and sulfur.
Protein atoms are huge, complex elements made by at least one wound and collapsed strands of amino acids. Proteins are amazingly confounded atoms that are effectively engaged with the most fundamental and significant pieces of life. These incorporate digestion, versatility,

safeguard, cell correspondence, and sub-atomic acknowledgment.

Proteins are macromolecular polypeptides, that are extremely huge particles (macromolecules) comprised of a few amino acids bound to the peptides.

Elements of Proteins

Positive negative connections between unmistakable molecules in the long amino corrosive strand make it curl on itself over and over to foster its profoundly convoluted shape. Collapsed proteins might get together with other collapsed proteins to produce considerably bigger, more complex structures.

The collapsed type of a protein particle directs its job in body science. Primary proteins are framed in manners that permit them to assemble basic designs of the body.

Collagen, a protein with a fiber structure, holds the greater part of the body tissues together. Keratin, one more underlying protein, delivers an organization of waterproof strands in the external layer of the skin.

Practical proteins have structures that empower them to partake in the substance cycles of the body. Practical proteins incorporate a portion of the chemicals, development factors, cell layer receptors, and catalysts.

Grouping of Proteins
Protein particles are large, complex substances made by at least one curved and collapsed strand of amino acids. Every amino corrosive is connected with the following amino corrosive through covalent bonds.

Essential (first level) - Protein structure is a grouping of amino acids in a chain.
Optional (auxiliary level) - Protein structure is produced by collapsing and contorting the amino corrosive chain.

Tertiary (third level) - Protein structure is created when the turns and overlap of the optional design overlay again to frame a greater three-layered structure.

Quaternary (fourth level) - Protein structure is a protein consisting of more than one collapsed amino corrosive chain.

Proteins can tie with other synthetic parts and structure "blended" atoms. For instance, glycoproteins secured in cell layers are proteins with sugars joined. Lipoproteins are lipid-protein combos.

Nucleic Acids

The two kinds of nucleic corrosive are deoxyribonucleic corrosive and ribonucleic corrosive. The fundamental structural units of nucleic acids are called nucleotides. Every nucleotide comprises a phosphate unit, a sugar, and a nitrogen base. DNA nucleotide bases incorporate adenine, thymine, guanine, and cytosine. RNA utilizes the indistinguishable succession of nucleotides, except for the trade of unit cells for thymine.

Nucleotides tie to each other to frame strands or different designs. In the DNA particle, nucleotides are coordinated and contorted, delivering a twofold strand called a twofold helix. The arrangement of different nucleotides along the DNA twofold helix is the "ace code" for building proteins and other nucleic acids.

Starches: The key occupation of sugar is to give energy and fuel the body the same way gas energizes a car. Food sources like , bread, cereal,plantains, rice, pasta, vegetables like potatoes ,peas ,corn,fruits and natural products give sugars or starches that give carbs for energy.

Energy assists the body with achieving day-to-day activities as basic as strolling and talking and as modern as running and moving enormous articles. Sustenance is required for development, which makes adequate food prominently basic for developing young people and expectant mothers Indeed, even very still, the body needs calories to achieve significant cycles, for example, keeping up with internal heat levels, keeping the heart thumping, and processing feasts.

What are sugars?
Carb is an assortment of compound substances present in natural tissues and food varieties such as starch, cellulose, and sucrose. The proportion of oxygen and hydrogen in carbs is equivalent to that of water for example 2:1. It typically separates in the creature's body to deliver energy.
Initially, the name sugar was utilized to indicate substances that were as a matter of fact "carbs," because they had the experimental recipe CH_2O. Starches have been arranged lately, founded on carb structures, not their formulae. Such aldehydes and ketones are currently perceived as polyhydroxy. Cellulose, starch,

and glycogen are among the substances that have a place in this family.

Carbs are additionally called sugars as a rule, certain to some extent methylated sugars and amino sugars normally and one regular nitro sugar is known. All sugars are polyhydroxy aldehydes or ketones or mixtures that create them on hydrolysis.

Sorts of Carbohydrates
-Straightforward Carbohydrates
Straightforward sugars are the basic type of carbs. Delicate drinks, sweets, treats, and other sweet treats incorporate straightforward carbs. These dishes are regularly delivered utilizing white sugar, a sort of handled sugar.

Straightforward carbs likewise are tracked down in normal sugars. Organic products, fruits and vegetables contain normal sugars. Honey is a characteristic sugar too. Individuals eat regular sugar in its unique structure. Straightforward sugars are more straightforward to deal with because they are less (or easier) complex. They begin from products of the soil things, as well as basically whatever else that is sweet. The human body can quickly separate these materials, and there is where a portion of the troubles lie.

There is only one sugar unit in the monosaccharides, subsequently, they are the littlest of the starches. "

The little size of monosaccharides bears the cost of them a particular job in processing and digestion. Before they can be eaten into the gastrointestinal plot, dietary carbs must be separated into monosaccharides and they additionally stream into monosaccharide structure in the blood.

- Complex Carbohydrates
Complex carbs give an indispensable energy source to your body. They give the supported sustenance your body needs for work out, day-to-day existence assignments, and even sleep.

Complex sugars are habitually single units (monosaccharides), which are fortified together. The oligosaccharides involve two to ten straightforward units of sugar. Polysaccharides involve hundreds and thousands of monosaccharides that are connected. Complex carbs have genuinely enduring energy.

The many types of starches can be ordered because of their conduct in hydrolysis. They are normally arranged into three gatherings:

Monosaccharides
Disaccharides
Polysaccharides

1. Monosaccharides
Monosaccharide starches are those carbs that can't be processed further to yield more straightforward units of polyhydroxy aldehyde or ketone. If a monosaccharide contains an aldehyde bunch, it is named aldose, and then again, if it contains a keto bunch, it is known as a ketose.

Functions

Monosaccharides are straightforwardly consumed by the small digestive system into the bloodstream,where they are moved to the cells out of luck. A few chemicals, including insulin and glucagon,are likewise part of the stomach related framework. They keep up with our glucose levels by eliminating or adding glucose to the circulation system on a case by case basis.

Monosaccharides in the body are energy stockpiling and as the structure blocks of additional mind boggling sugars that are utilized as primary components. Monosaccharides are glasslike solids that are dissolvable in water, and typically have a sweet taste.

Instances of monosaccharides : oats, barbecue,wheat, Apples, banana strawberry,grapes.

- Glucose

One of the main monosaccharides is glucose. The two for the most part used strategies for the creation of glucose are

From Sucrose: If sucrose is cooked with weak corrosive in a heavy drinker arrangement then we get glucose and fructose.

From Starch: We can acquire glucose by hydrolysis of starch .

Glucose is likewise named aldohexose and dextrose and is plentiful on the planet.

The ring construction of glucose makes sense of numerous parts of glucose that can't be figured out by an open-chain structure.

The two cyclic designs contrast in the game plan of the hydroxyl bunch at C_1 called anomeric carbon. Such isomers for example α and β structures are known as anomers.

The cyclic design is now and again called pyranose structure in light of its likeness with pyran.

- Fructose

It is a significant ketohexose and has a ketone practical gathering and includes six carbon iotas.

The ring part of fructose is in relationship to the compound Furan and is named furanose.

2. Disaccharides

On hydrolysis, disaccharides produce two atoms of either the equivalent or various monosaccharides.

The two monosaccharide units are associated with oxide linkage which is made by the deficiency of water particles and this linkage is called glycosidic linkage.

Sucrose is the most regular disaccharide that on hydrolysis creates glucose and fructose.

Maltose and Lactose (otherwise called milk sugar) are the other two significant disaccharides.

In maltose, there are two α-D-glucose

also, in lactose, there are two B-D-glucose Function

Keeps a sound body, gives the body glucose which gives energy. It assists with building particles like proteins and lipids. Disaccharides assists in the retention of different supplements with preferring nutrients and minerals.
Food sources : natural products like mango, orange, banana, berries, pawpaw, watermelon.
vegetables: carrot, lentils, spinach, lettuce.
Sodas and table sugar are associated by an oxide association

3 Polysaccharides: Polysaccharides contain extended monosaccharide units connected by glycosidic linkage.
The greater part of them goes about as food stockpiling for example Starch. Starch is the primary stockpiling polysaccharide for plants.
It is a polymer of α glucose and comprises two parts Amylose and Amylopectin.

Cellulose is additionally one of the polysaccharides that are normally tracked down in plants.

It is shaped by β-D-glucose units associated with a glycosidic connection between C_1 of one glucose unit and C_4 of the following glucose unit.

Functions: Polysaccharides give underlying support, store energy, and convey cell correspondence messages.

Food sources:
Cornmeal, oats, rice, millet, pasta, unripe natural products.

What sort of food sources are starches?
Carbs are available in a great many protected as well as unfortunate food varieties (processed foods) such as beans, sorghum, potatoes, pasta, barley, wheat, rice corn, cereal.

They arrive in a scope of shapes as well. The most normal and bountiful structures are sugars, carbs, and filaments.

What are the significant jobs of carbs?
The four fundamental carb jobs in the body are to create energy, store energy, produce macromolecules, and extra protein and fat for different necessities. Glucose energy is utilized as glycogen, with most in the muscle and liver.

What are the principal starches?
Food varieties rich in carbs incorporate bread, vegetables, and organic products, as well as dairy. Carbs are the sugars, starches, and strands present in the results of natural products, grains, vegetables, and milk. Although frequently defamed in popular weight control plans, starches are crucial for a sound eating regimen as one of the essential nutritional categories.

What are the two wellsprings of carbs?
Sound starch sources incorporate both creatures and plant dietary sources, like new natural products, tomatoes, corn, potatoes,

meat, and milk items. Models that are undependable incorporate pop, white bread, added sugar, baked goods, and other profoundly handled feasts.

What is straightforward sugar?
The body quickly separates basic carbs to be utilized as energy. Straightforward carbs are normally found in dinners like organic products, milk, and dairy items. Handled and refined sugars like sugar beets, table sugar, syrups, and glucose, are additionally found.

What is an intricate starch?
Straightforward starches comprise sugar atoms, which are bound together in lengthy, complex chains. Food sources like peas, beans, entire grains, and vegetables incorporate complex carbs. Inside the body, both basic and complex carbs are changed into glucose (glucose) and utilized as energy.

What is the contrast between intricate and straightforward sugars?

Straightforward starches are available in such dinners as table sugar and syrups. Complex carbs incorporate longer sugar atom chains than conventional carbs. Since complex carbs have longer chains, they take more time than straightforward starches to separate and give seriously enduring energy to the body.

Fat: Dietary fat, which is tracked down in oils, coconut, nuts, milk, cheddar, meat, chicken, and fish, gives design to cells and pads layers to assist with forestalling harm. Oils and fats are likewise expected for retaining fat-dissolvable nutrients including vitamin A, a substance significant for solid eyes and lungs.

Dietary fat is an energy-thick supplement that conveys significant unsaturated fats (FAs) and helps in fat-dissolvable nutrient assimilation. At the point when dietary fat retention becomes dysregulated, it adds to adjusted blood lipid levels and metabolic illness risk. Triacylglycerol (TAG), the essential kind of dietary fat, is immediately retained (>93%). Its assimilation items are taken up by enterocytes, the absorptive cells of the small digestive system, and quickly resynthesized into TAG. This resynthesized TAG is either integrated into chylomicrons (CMs) and emitted into dissemination through lymph for conveyance to fringe tissues or integrated into cytoplasmic lipid drops (CLDs) . On the other hand, absorption results of dietary fat may likewise be incorporated into additional complicated lipids, go about as flagging atoms, or act as an energy source.

Dietary fat is processed and consumed in the small digestive tract and can hence be utilized as an energy source or potentially as a supply for other bioactive lipid particles. Exorbitant dietary fat has been connected to the acceptance as well as compounding of different issues, including colorectal malignant growth (CRC). Abstains from food with the high-fat substance have been shown to demolish CRC through regulation of digestive irritation and expansion, as well as change of bile corrosive pools, microbiota, and bioactive lipid specie

Micronutrition: Vitamins and Minerals

Nutrients help in energy creation, wound recuperating, bone structure, resistance, and eye and skin wellbeing.

Minerals assist with saving cardiovascular wellbeing and proposition design to the skeleton.

Devouring a decent eating routine with natural products, vegetables, dairy, protein food sources, and entire or improved grains guarantees the body has a lot of supplements to utilize. Giving a couple of instances of explicit micronutrient capabilities can improve the viability of sustenance training:

Vitamin A assists the eyes with seeing

Calcium and magnesium help muscles and veins unwind, decreasing squeezing and hypertension

L-ascorbic acid assists wounds with mending and the body's capacity to battle against contaminations

Iron assists the blood with moving oxygen all through the body and forestalls paleness

Nutrients and minerals are micronutrients expected by the body to do a scope of normal errands. Nonetheless, these micronutrients are not made in our bodies and should be taken from the food we eat.

Nutrients are natural atoms that are typically classed as either fat dissolvable or water-solvent. Fat-solvent nutrients (vitamin A, vitamin D, vitamin E, and vitamin K) break up in fat and will more often than not gather in the body. Water-solvent nutrients (L-ascorbic acid and the B-complex nutrients, like vitamin B6, vitamin B12, and folate) should disintegrate in water before they can be consumed by the body, and thus can't be reserved in the body .Any water-solvent nutrients unused by the body are generally lost through pee.

Minerals: minerals in food are the constituents encompassed in the food that is needed by our body to mature and work appropriately."

Minerals in food:
What are Minerals and why are they important? From the above definition, we might establish that minerals are inorganic mixtures essential for the human body to work accurately . The human body requires fluctuating measures of minerals every day to deliver solid bones and muscles. It likewise assists with supporting various natural capabilities. Thus, we get these supplements by utilizing and eating meals opulent in minerals.
At the point when the body doesn't obtain an adequate number of minerals, this could

lead to enervating illnesses such as pellagra, scurvy, Anemia, Rickets, Hypocalcemia.

Examples of Minerals foods:
There are different sources of minerals in food; these include:
Chloride
Magnesium
Zinc
Sodium and iron

Sustenance:
Sustenance is what food means for the strength of the body.
Sustenance is a pivotal component of a sound way of life and the significance of getting it appropriately can't be worried - we should begin by jumping into the advantages of having a nutritious eating routine.

How fantastic nourishment build your well-being

• Weight control

A ton of us wrongly interface weight reduction with trend counts calories, yet eating a nutritious feast is the best way to deal with the approach of keeping a sound weight and simultaneously getting the important supplements for the ideal physical process. Trading unfortunate low-quality food and bites out for nutritious food is the initial step to keeping your weight inside a sound reach as indicated by your body organization, without the need to get on board with the craze diet fad.

• Safeguarding you from constant issues

Numerous persistent infections, for example, type-2 diabetes and coronary illness are initiated by less than stellar eating routine and weight. With 1 out of 9 Americans experiencing diabetes, the accentuation on sufficient eating is higher than at any other time. Adopting a preventive strategy with an entire food-based nourishment plan likewise limits the gamble of gaining other related problems like kidney disappointment.

- Reinforcing your unsusceptible framework

Our invulnerable framework requires basic nutrients and minerals to proficiently work. Eating a decent and various eating routine ensures your invulnerable framework performs at max execution and prepares for diseases and immunodeficiency problems.

- Deferring the beginning of maturing (anti-ageing)

Specific sorts of food, for example, papaya,blueberries,spinach,Broccoli,can increment imperativeness and work on mental execution, meanwhile defending your body against the outcomes of maturing.(ageing)

- Supporting your psychological prosperity

Eating suitable food varieties can make you more joyful — minerals, for example, iron and omega-3 unsaturated fats present in a protein-rich eating routine can expand your temperament. This serves to higher generally speaking mental prosperity and safeguards you against psychological well-being issues.

All in all, how can one foster a sensible eating routine arrangement then, at that point? Good dieting is tied in with devouring adjusted extents of supplement-rich food varieties from the significant nutrition classes, as well as following specific good dieting ways of behaving.

The most effective method to get satisfactory nourishment in your eating routine
Every nutritional category contains unmistakable supplements and benefits, in this manner eating a fair eating regimen

that incorporates food sources from each of the five gatherings is essential. These are the different nutritional categories that you ought to remember.

1. Entire grains

Entire grain food sources, for example, earthy colored rice and bread are sorts of carbs, explicitly raw carbs. They supply you with energy, solid fiber, nutrients, minerals, and cancer prevention agents, and help with assimilation. For people who are determined to have coeliacs or those with non-coeliac gluten responsiveness, you should incorporate other carb choices to guarantee that your restraint from wheat doesn't cost you key supplements.

2. Products of the soil

Different sorts of these items are great suppliers of nutrients and minerals that help control the body working and safeguard it against ongoing afflictions. To get the most supplements out of your products of the soil, eat them entirely - for instance polish off whole natural products as opposed to having squeezed seapods, tomatoes, pumpkins, cucumbers .

3. Protein
Protein is the key food answerable for making and fixing muscle tissue in the body. Creature meat is the most predominant wellspring of protein, however, there are additionally different plant-based sources to pick from like nuts and vegetables. People on plant-based diets ought to guarantee they eat the appropriate blend of plant protein to guarantee that their dietary requests are adequatcly tended to.

4. Dairy
Dairy items are plentiful in imperative minerals like calcium, potassium, sodium,and nutrients A, D, and B2. Food sources like cheese, yogurt, butter,and ice cream, are awesome instances of dairy

which can be bought in virtually every supermarket.

5. Fat and sugar

Dietary fat, for example, the sort you get from fish and olive oil is fundamental for ideal wellbeing as they oversee cholesterol levels in your body while supporting sound cell action. Monounsaturated, polyunsaturated, and immersed fat all have a section in this component of ideal wellbeing. Then again, the extra fat you normally find in broiled food ought to be restricted as they are generally polyunsaturated fat gotten from handled vegetable oils like soybean and sunflower

Because of their low edge for oxidization, overconsumption of polyunsaturated fat can prompt fiery circumstances and the age of free revolutionaries. Fake trans fat is likewise a severe "no". Sugar ought to likewise be controlled — while the normal sugars accessible in foods grown from the ground grains are valuable, the refined assortment you get with cakes and tidbits can change your weight and add to metabolic diseases whenever ingested in overabundance.

Aside from eating dinners from the previously mentioned nutritional categories, there are three more smart dieting propensities to keep up with to keep your sustenance anticipate point.

• Keep segment sums limited
Overseeing segment sizes is tied in with guaranteeing that you are getting the legitimate measures of supplements and calories from your eating regimen. Gorging or under-eating denies you supplements and could influence your weight, so consistently control your feast amounts. While purchasing food, pay special attention to the serving sizes on the nourishment marks to

see what compares to a standard serving and the amount it conveys regarding supplements.

• Focus on new food
New, entire food varieties are the ones you will acquire the best wholesome advantages from. Continuously go for things in their most flawless, pure structure like new organic products, vegetables, and meat when possible. Assuming you go with handled other options, consider those that have gone through minor adjustments like drying out and streak freezing to lessen supplement misfortune. Additionally, watch out for the fixings rundown to guarantee that you're taking a couple of added substances with your food as could be expected.

• Pursue solid flavoring routines
Think about offsetting your salt admission with different spices and flavors to offer another layer of taste to your food. For

instance, shallot,garlic,leek, and onions can transform a standard turkey bosom dish into a gastronomic treat! Salt is the most well-known food preparation utilized in cooking, however, an excessive amount of sodium can prompt hypertension, especially in people who are as of now defenseless to said conditions.

Keeping a nutritious eating plan is sufficiently basic; breaking down whether it's nutritious enough can be clear too. Simply pay special attention to five fundamental enough markers of whether you are getting enough from your food.

Marks of an invigorating eating routine

1. Body arrangement
A very organized nourishment plan ought to permit a person to keep a sound build inside This additionally implies that it ought to help metabolic wellbeing through a few systems, for example, supporting solid

chemical capability, insulin responsiveness, and actual recuperation.

2. Solid cholesterol levels and pulse
Observing your cholesterol levels and pulse is essential because having a solid weight doesn't lessen the probability of entanglements in these regions. While dietary cholesterol doesn't affect blood cholesterol levels as we previously accepted, it can in any case be impacted by your general dietary fat admission. Then again, high salt admission can prompt hypertension, of which one of the side effects is raised pulse levels.

3. Solid skin and hair
The condition of your skin and hair are dependable marks of the nature of your nourishment. If you are getting sufficient supplements, your skin ought to be firm, versatile, and of a rich tone as opposed to

flaky and colorless. Your hair ought to be velvety and vigorous instead of dry and weak; unexplained balding is by and large a sign of starvation.

4. Rest and energy levels
Getting a legitimate number of supplements and calories will assist you with remaining fortified because of its ability to help serene rest. On the off chance that you discover yourself feeling lazy, It could be an indication of either a particular absence of calories as well as supplements, driving your body into "starvation mode" which restricts its fixing powers.

5. Customary inside movements
Your entrail movements demonstrate whether you are getting adequate fiber from your eating routine, so assuming you regard yourself as becoming obstructed, top off on additional leafy foods to get your stomach-related framework streaming.

Chapter 2

The Influence of diet on Health

The food we eat gives our bodies the "data" and parts they expect to work. On the off chance that we don't get the right data, our metabolic situation disintegrates, and our wellbeing declines.

Assuming we get an excessive amount of food or food that sends our bodies some unacceptable guidelines, we could become overweight, undernourished, and at risk for the improvement of illnesses and issues, like joint pain, diabetes, and coronary illness.

In outline, what we eat is vital to our wellbeing.

Food capabilities as medication — to maintain, forestall, and treat sickness.

What does food do in our bodies?

The supplements in food empower the cells in our body to satisfy their crucial positions...

"Supplements are the supporting parts in food that are expected for the development, improvement, and upkeep of physiological capabilities. That is ,intending on the off chance that a supplement isn't there, parts of capability and thus human wellbeing reduce. At the point when nourishment admission doesn't consistently match the supplement needs expected by the cell movement, the metabolic exercises are delayed or even stop.

At the end of the day, supplements give our bodies guidelines about how to work. In this regard, food can be viewed as a wellspring of "information" for the body.

Contemplating food in this manner gives us a dream of nourishment that stretches out past calories or grams, great food sources, or unfortunate dinners. This mentality makes us center around things we ought to incorporate instead of ones to avoid.

Rather than seeing food as the enemy, we shift focus over to food as a strategy to make well-being and forestall disorder by assisting the body with supporting capability.

What is a portion of the worries with our eating regimen?

Handling takes out sustenance

Our grocery stores are brimming with simple bundled dinners that entice your taste buds but weaken our nourishment. Since a large portion of these food sources' inborn supplements are disposed of in the refining system, handled food sources have accession.

Our Standard American Diet depends fundamentally on handled food sources that incorporate counterfeit tone, added substances, flavorings, and artificially modified fats and sugars. These synthetic compounds and artificially changed substances might be giving our bodies some unacceptable signs, rather than the data they need to successfully work.

Indeed "regular" feasts have fewer supplements

Our food isn't equivalent to what it was a long time back. Supplements in the ground have been exhausted, consequently, food developed in that ground has fewer supplements. Synthetic substances are progressively utilized in creating the two plants and animals, especially on enormous modern homesteads that have some expertise in a couple of products.

We are eating less assortment of feasts. Incidentally, while 16000 new things are fostered every year, 66% of our calories begin from only four food sources: corn, soy, wheat, and rice.

We eat for comfort, not joy. We will more often than not consume for comfort and speed, not wellbeing and happiness. Our quick food varieties likewise divert us from the delights of making and valuing a wonderful dinner,

What is the association between food and illness?
As a general public, we are encountering serious well-being challenges.
The United States positions 10th in the future among countries in the created world. We have a labor force burdened with truancy and unfortunate efficiency in light of the persistent medical issue, including misery.
75% of medical care costs are for the therapy of persistent illness.
Many examinations currently feel that these problems are incompletely connected with food. While specialists used to accept that illnesses like sort II diabetes, stoutness, coronary illness, stroke, and a few malignancies - were brought about by **a** solitary quality change, they are present, by and large, crediting these illnesses to an organization of cell glitch. What's more, the

food we eat is a significant component in that brokenness, to a limited extent because our weight control plans miss the mark on the legitimate equilibrium of supplements.

To forestall the development of these illnesses, we want to get a handle on what various supplements in an eating routine cooperate and mean for the human body's exercises, as per the Nutrition Society, . Utilitarian Medicine is a unique strategy for evaluating, forestalling, and treating intricate and ongoing illnesses using nourishment. This part of medical care likewise concentrates on the impact that diet plays on wellbeing.

The Utilitarian medical Perspective
Human stomach-related framework One part of Utilitarian Medicine centers around what eating means for wellbeing and capability. At the point when Utilitarian Medicine specialists investigate the job of sustenance in ongoing illness, they take a

gander at numerous frameworks, like the stomach-related framework, the immunological framework, and the detoxification framework, due to the interconnections between those frameworks. For example, because 75% of the resistant framework is contained in the gastrointestinal plot, an individual's issues with invulnerability could be attached to ill-advised processing.

Useful Medicine holds that constant illness is almost perpetually gone before by a time of decreasing wellbeing in at least one of the body's frameworks. In this way, these experts endeavor to find early the signs that signal hidden brokenness, conceivably prompting illness.

One of the manners in which Utilitarian Medicine expects to treat bombing wellbeing is to give the feasts and supplements expected to reestablish capability. This is a savvy, harmless method that attempts to capture the movement into disease.

Illustration of Cardiovascular Disease

While adopting a dietary strategy for wellbeing and infection, it is significant to recollect that one sickness could have a few beginnings, and one hidden ailment could cause various illnesses. Cardiovascular sickness might be among the clearest instances of this thought.

Scientists have uncovered that the advancement of cardiovascular illness can be set off by different factors. These elements incorporate insulin opposition, high homocysteine, oxidative pressure, raised cholesterol, hypertension, weighty metal poisonousness, stress, and irritation. Every one of these components can be constrained by sustenance and each, thus, influences our nourishing requests. This applies both to the anticipation and treatment of these issues.

Chapter 3

Overweight (Types, causes, treatment, and prevention)

What is obesity?
Stoutness is a perplexing, constant condition with different variables that lead to unnecessary muscle versus fat and of time, chronic weakness. Muscle-to-fat ratio itself isn't an ailment. Yet, when your body has an excessive amount of extra fat, it could influence how it works. These adjustments are moderate, can deteriorate over the long run, and they can prompt critical well-being results.

Fortunately, you can further develop your well-being gambles by shedding some portion of your abundance of muscle versus fat. Indeed, even minuscule changes in weight can impact your wellbeing. Few out of every odd weight reduction approach works for everybody. A great many people have attempted to decrease weight at least a time or two. What's more, keeping the load off is similarly basically as vital as losing it in any case.

Is stoutness portrayed by your weight?
Medical practitioners frequently use the Body Mass Index (BMI) to characterize stoutness in everybody. The BMI estimates normal body weight versus normal body level. As speculation, medical practitioners liken a BMI of 30 or above to corpulence. Although BMI has its impediments, it's an effectively quantifiable measurement and can assist with making you aware of corpulence-related medical issues.

Instances of limitations are jocks and competitors, who have more muscle and may have higher BMI scores even while their fat levels are unassuming. It's likewise conceivable to have corpulence at an "ordinary" weight. On the off chance that your body weight is normal however your muscle versus fat ratio is high, you might have similar well-being gambles as someone with a higher BMI.

Medical practitioners have likewise found ethnic fluctuations in how much extra weight different individuals might convey before it influences their wellbeing. For instance, individuals of Asian plunge individuals are bound to have well-being gambles at a lower BMI, and Black individuals are bound to have well-being and take a chance at a higher BMI.

One more approach to surveying corpulence is by estimating the midsection perimeter. Assuming you have more muscle versus fat around your midsection, you are measurably more in danger of stoutness-related illnesses. The gamble becomes huge when your midsection size is more than 35 creeps for individuals appointed female upon entering the world or 40 crawls for individuals allocated male upon entering the world.

What are the three classes of corpulence?
Medical services specialists characterize weight into different kinds in light of how serious it is. They utilize BMI to make it happen. On the off chance that your BMI is somewhere in the range of 25 and 29.9 they put you in the overweight class. There are three expansive sorts of weight that medical care specialists use to assess what treatments might turn out best for every individual. They include:

Class I corpulence: BMI 30 to <35 kg/m².
Class II corpulence: BMI 35 to <40 kg/m².
Class III corpulence: BMI 40+ kg/m².

What is "bleak" stoutness?
"Grim stoutness" is an old name for class III corpulence. In clinical language, "grimness" signifies connected well-being concerns. Specialists alluded to class III corpulence as "sullen" since it was probably going to accompany connected wellbeing concerns.

Be that as it may, they stopped the name because of its negative ramifications.

How is youth weight evaluated?
Medical practitioners additionally use BMI to decide corpulence in youngsters, however, they register it as connected with the kid's age and relegated sex. A kid more established than 2 years might be determined to have stoutness on the off chance that their BMI is more prominent than 95% of their companions in a similar gathering. Different development diagrams might give marginally various BMI midpoints, reliant upon the populace they are inspecting.

How continuous is stoutness?
Corpulence in American grown-ups was last overviewed in 2018. The recurrence was 42%, up from 30.% in 1999-2000. In that equivalent period, the commonness of class III corpulence practically multiplied from

4.7% to 8.2%. Adolescence stoutness in America ranges from 18.4%- 20.9%.

Around the world, corpulence has generally significantly increased in the past 50 years. The flood has been particularly striking in lower-pay nations where a lack of healthy sustenance is endemic. These people groups currently have expanded admittance to more unhealthy things with fewer health benefits. Corpulence presently consistently exists together with undernutrition in these nations.

Side effects and causes

How in all actuality does fat impact my body?

Corpulence influences your body in different ways. Some are only the mechanical impacts of having an additional muscle-to-fat ratio. For instance, you can define an unmistakable boundary between expanded load on your body and additional strain on your skeleton and joints. Different effects are more unpretentious, like substance changes in your blood that increment your gamble for diabetes, coronary illness, and stroke.

A few effects are as yet not perceived. For instance, there is an expanded gamble of specific malignancies with weight. We don't have the foggiest idea why, yet it exists. Genuinely, corpulence raises the gamble of unexpected precocious passing from all causes. All the same, concentrate on demonstrating the way that you can emphatically work on these dangers by dropping even a minor measure of weight (5% to 10%).

Metabolic changes

Your digestion is the method involved with switching food into energy completely to fuel your body's capabilities. At the point when your body has a larger number of calories than it can require, it transforms the extra calories into lipids and stores them in your fat tissue (muscle to fat ratio). At the point when you run out of tissue to store lipids in, the fat cells themselves get bigger. Broadened fat cells emit chemicals and different synthetics that produce a provocative reaction.

Persistent irritation has a few unfavorable well-being suggestions. One way that it influences your digestion is by adding to insulin opposition. This implies your body can never again utilize insulin to productively bring down blood glucose and blood lipid levels (sugars and fats in your blood). High glucose and blood lipids (cholesterol and fatty oils) likewise add to hypertension.

Together, these joined gambling factors are known as metabolic conditions. They are assembled because they generally will more often than not build up one another. They additionally support further weight gain and make it harder to get in shape and support weight reduction. Metabolic condition is typically considered stoutness and adds to many related infections, including:

Type 2 diabetes. Weight explicitly raises the gamble of Type 2 diabetes seven-increase in individuals allocated male upon entering the world and a 12-overlay in individuals relegated female upon entering the world. The gamble accelerates by 20% for each extra point you gain on the BMI scale. It additionally lessens with weight reduction. Cardiovascular illness: Hypertension, elevated cholesterol, high glucose, and irritation are all hazard factors for cardiovascular illnesses, including coronary conduit illness, congestive cardiovascular breakdown, respiratory failure, and stroke. These dangers escalate together with your BMI. Cardiovascular illness is the main source of preventable demise overall and in the U.S. Fatty liver sickness. The abundance of fats flowing in your blood advance toward your liver, which is answerable for sifting your blood. At the point when your liver starts putting away an overabundance of fat, it can prompt ongoing liver irritation (hepatitis) and long haul liver harm (cirrhosis) (cirrhosis).

Kidney illness: High pulse, diabetes, and liver sickness are among the most widely recognized supporters of persistent kidney infection.

Gallstones. Higher blood cholesterol levels can make cholesterol aggregate in your gallbladder, prompting cholesterol gallstones and potential gallbladder illnesses.

Direct impacts

An abundance of muscle versus fat can swarm the organs of your respiratory framework and put pressure and burden on your outer muscle framework. This adds to:

Asthma.

Rest apnea.

Obesity hypoventilation syndrome.

Osteoarthritis.

Backache.

According to the U.S. Centers for Disease Control and Prevention, 1 in 4 persons with obesity also has arthritis. Studies have found that for every 5 kg in weight gain, your risk of knee arthritis increases by 33%. The good news is that, along with exercise, weight loss of 10% can dramatically reduce arthritis-related discomfort and enhance your quality of life.

Indirect effects
Obesity is also connected indirectly with:
Memory and cognition, including a heightened risk of Alzheimer's disease and dementia.
Female infertility and pregnancy problems.
Depression and mood disorders.
Certain malignancies include esophageal, pancreatic, colorectal, breast, uterine, and ovarian.

What causes obesity?
On the most basic level, obesity is caused by consuming more calories than your body can utilize. Many variables contribute to this. Some elements are particular to you. Others are built into the structure of our society, either on a national, local, or family level. In some ways, preventing obesity entails intentionally working against these numerous causes.

Factors that may increase calorie consumption include:
Fast and convenient foods. In communities and households where highly-processed fast and convenience meals are dietary staples, it's simple to consume a lot of calories. These foods are high in sugar and fat and poor in fiber and other nutrients, which can make you hungry. Their components induce addictive eating tendencies. In some places, these may be the only sorts of foods easily available, due to both cost and access. The Centers for Disease Control estimate that

43% of households in America reside more than a mile from healthy food retailers.

Sugar is in everything. The food sector is not meant to sustain our health. It's designed to market items that we will become addicted to and want to buy more of. High on that list of products are sweets and sugary drinks, which have no nutritious value and a lot of extra calories. But even normal foods have large levels of added sugar to make them more tempting and addicting. It's so widespread that it's transformed our taste expectations.

Marketing and advertising: Pervasive advertising pushes processed foods, sweets, and sugary\drinks, the items that we need the least but that the industry wants us to buy the most. Advertising makes these products seem like a normal and necessary part of everyday life. Advertising also plays a big part in selling alcoholic drinks, which add a lot of empty calories.

Psychological aspects:

Boredom, loneliness, anxiety, and depression are all common in modern society, and can all lead to overeating. They may specifically lead to eating certain sorts of meals that activate pleasure centers in our brains, foods that tend to be higher in calories. Eating to feel better is a natural human instinct. We evolved to locate food, and evolution hasn't caught up to the kind of availability of food that Western civilizations currently enjoy.

Hormones:

Hormones influence our hunger and satiety signals. Many things can disrupt these regulatory processes, including common things like stress and lack of sleep and less common things like genetic variations. Hormones can cause you to continue to crave more food even when you don't need any more calories. They can make it hard to recognize when you've had enough.

Certain medications:
Medications that you take to address other problems may lead to weight gain. Antidepressants, steroids, cardiovascular medications, diabetes medications, are among them.

Factors that may decrease how many calories we extend to include:
Screen culture: As work, shopping and social life continue to move online, we progressively spend more time in front of our phones and computers. Streaming media and binge-watching make long hours of sedentary entertainment more possible.

Workforce changes: With industry shifts going toward automation and technology, more employees today work at desks than on their feet. They also work longer hours.

Fatigue: Sedentary lifestyles have a snowball effect. Studies show that the longer you sit still, the wearier and less motivated you become. Sitting makes your body stiff and contributes to aches and pains that discourage movement. It also causes general stress, which adds to fatigue.

Neighborhood design:
Many people lack local places to be active, either due to access or safety issues. More than half of Americans don't live within half a mile of a park. They may not live in walkable neighborhoods, and they may not see others in their communities being active in day-to-day living. When there is no public transportation alternative, most individuals can only commute by automobile.

Childcare trends: Children spend less time playing outside than they used to. They spend more time in enclosed daycare spaces, which may not offer appropriate rooms or facilities for physical activity. This is partly due to cultural trends that don't find it safe for children to play outside unattended. It's also due to inadequate access to public spaces and inadequate access to quality childcare. Many childcare environments substitute TV for free play.

Disability: Adults and children with physical and learning disabilities are particularly at risk for obesity. Physical restrictions and lack of proper specialist knowledge and resources can contribute.

DIAGNOSIS AND TESTS
How is obesity diagnosed?
Your healthcare provider will measure your weight, height, and waist circumference at your appointment.
More importantly, when you come to your healthcare provider for care, they will want to know your full health narrative. They will get some information about your set of experiences of clinical issues, prescriptions, and weight changes. They'll likewise need to find out about your ongoing eating, resting, and action practices and stress elements and whether you have endeavored any health

improvement plans previously. They might scrutinize your natural family's well-being history.

They will likewise survey your essential capabilities by taking your pulse and circulatory strain and paying attention to your heart and lungs. They might give you a blood test to evaluate your blood glucose and cholesterol levels and screen for chemical irregularities. They'll use this complete profile to recognize your corpulence and any connected ailments you could have.

THE BOARD AND TREATMENT
How is corpulence treated?
Your whole well-being profile will lay out your particular treatment approach. Your medical services proficiency will focus on your most dire wellbeing concerns first, then, at that point, circle back to a more extended-term weight reduction plan. In some cases, there might be quick alterations they can suggest for a moment's influence,

such as changing your meds. The absolute treatment approach will be more continuous and possibly involve various angles. Since everybody is unique, it might take experimentation to sort out which treatments turn out best for you. Studies have more than once shown that forceful, group-based programs with regular, individual correspondence between your doctor and you are the most advantageous in assisting individuals with shedding pounds and keeping it off.

Your treatment technique might include:
Dietary changes:
The dietary alterations you need to make to get in shape will be specific to you. Certain individuals might profit from bringing down segment sums or nibbling between dinners. For other people, it very well might be more about adjusting what they eat than how much. Nearly everybody can profit from eating more plants. Organic products, vegetables, entire grains, and vegetables will

quite often be lower in fat and higher in fiber and micronutrients. They are more nutritious and could cause you to feel more full and more satisfied after eating fewer calories.

Expanded movement:
Everybody has heard that food and exercise are both fundamental to weight reduction and weight upkeep. In any case, practicing doesn't need to mean a rec center enrollment. Simply strolling at a moderate speed is one of the most proficient techniques for practice for weight reduction. minimum of 35minutes, is required. A day-to-day stroll at noon or previously or after work can have a gigantic effect.

Anticipation
How might I forestall corpulence?
Forestalling weight is more straightforward than treating it whenever it has grabbed hold. When your body has been laid out Add a little movement. On the other hand, figure

out how you could spend an extra 155 calories in a day. For instance, go for a climb or utilize a curved machine for 30 minutes, or take the canine for a lively stroll for 40 minutes.

Shopping intentionally:
Stock your home with quality food varieties and save desserts and treats for extraordinary events when you go out. Entire food varieties are higher in fiber and lower on the glycemic file, so they don't cause your glucose to spike and drop like handled tidbits and treats do.

Develop generally speaking wellbeing:
Diminish your screen time, head outside, and take a walk. Deal with your pressure and attempt to get fitting rest to keep your chemical levels in line. Center around certain progressions and solid exercises instead of what your endeavors mean for your weight.

STANDPOINT/PROGNOSIS

What is the best future for me assuming I have corpulence?

Stoutness jeopardizes you with a few destructive medical problems. That doesn't mean you have those side effects at this moment. Also, it doesn't imply that you can't hope to make any significant difference either way. The dangers merit your concern, but at the same time, they're reversible or treatable. Your medical care practitioner will urge you to bring them down by diminishing weight. While it will be extreme, it can be achieved.

Keep in mind that weight reduction of only 6% to 10% can impressively further develop your well-being. It can diminish or stop the movement of greasy liver sickness, metabolic disorders, and diabetes. With clinical bearing, weight reduction of essentially this sum is achievable, and potentially extensively more. Staying with a drawn-out treatment plan can assist you with keeping up with weight reduction.

Chapter 4

Highly classified Eating Habits To Reverse Aging

1. Limit your utilization of unhealthy food:
One of the most settled upon procedures to help down your maturing interaction is diminishing your utilization of added sugar. Also, perhaps the most immediate way you can accomplish this is by limiting how much handled low-quality food you eat.

Eating a lot of low-quality food can prompt medical problems that can make significant challenges in the body, so to carry on with a long, solid life, consider keeping away from the enticement of unhealthy food like treats and cakes at whatever point you can.

2. Eat more greasy fish:
Integrating more fish into your eating regimen can upgrade your well-being in more ways than one, particularly as you progress in years. "Fish is brimming with omega-3 unsaturated fats, which can

safeguard your body from disorder," and omega-3 unsaturated fats help with heart issues, melancholy, and even malignant growth as you age."
On the off chance that you're not an admirer of eating fish, you may likewise profit from investigating taking some omega-3 pills all things considered.

3. Eat more beautiful products of the soil:
  eating a lot of leafy foods is a useful propensity in fighting the maturing system.
"Instances of valuable foods grown from the ground incorporate spinach, watercress, citrus, salads greens, carrots, and red pepper, since these are high in cell reinforcements and fiber, which offset the negative impacts of maturing;"(aging)"

4. Trade meat for plant-based protein:
In certain circumstances, restricting your meat admission and expanding your utilization of plant-based proteins like beans and lentils will assist you with slowly

bringing down the maturing system(aging). Adding more vegetables like spinach, lettuce Broccoli, celery, cabbage, into your dinners might diminish the maturing system by bringing down cholesterol levels, directing glucose, and decreasing aggravation. It's essential to in any case ensure you're eating a reasonable eating routine that matches your way of life.

5. Remain hydrated:
Perhaps the biggest age-related trouble that surfaces for some people is parchedness. As we age, numerous frameworks that we depend on to keep us hydrated start to corrupt, like the kidneys, and a few normal age-related medications can cause an expansion in water misfortune.
And keeping in mind that water is typically the best way for hydration, you may likewise add hydrating things to your everyday eating routine. "
A few food varieties can assist with advancing hydration like cucumbers,

cantaloupe, watermelon, tomatoes, strawberries, peaches Zucchini and oranges since these food sources have a high water content, which can help improve hydration while likewise contributing enemy of maturing cell reinforcement parts to the eating routine.

6. Pecans:

Pecans are a great multitasker with regards to life span. Ladies who ingested nuts, especially pecans, around midlife were bound to progress in years restoratively contrasted with the people who didn't eat nuts "Sound maturing" was characterized as having no constant illnesses, announced mental debilitation, and actual constraints, as well as having unblemished psychological well-being after the age of 60.

Pecans likewise have a fundamental capability in heart wellbeing. The principal research on cardiovascular wellbeing and pecans was distributed quite a while back in the New England Journal of Medicine, and since that time, there have been handfuls and many examinations on heart wellbeing, A meta-investigation of 24 preliminaries on heart wellbeing has demonstrated the way that pecans can bring down your all-out cholesterol and fatty oils, assist with controlling solid circulatory strain, and contain a lot of calming phytochemicals.In conclusion, mental wellbeing is significant to life span: Many examinations have shown that pecans and their synergistic supplements and phytochemicals — the omega-3 fats, fiber, protein, and polyphenols, in addition to different minerals and nutrients — may assist with deferring the start, lessen the advancement, and support mental capability as we age. This is a huge enemy of maturing objectives(anti ageing supplement) "We need to live well as well as live long, and mental wellbeing is critical".

7. Beans and Legumes:

Beans are one of few food sources that length two dietary classes: starches and protein. They're a major piece of the Mediterranean eating routine, which is one the best weight control plans and normal where individuals carry on with long and well residing.

Vegetables are a significant patron of plant-based protein and have been found to decrease the gamble of major ongoing infections and increase wellbeing and life span. They're stacked with phytonutrients, nutrients, minerals, fiber that helps the heart and digestive organs, glucose dependability, certain malignancies risk, solid weight control,

Beans are staggeringly flexible. lima, chickpeas, mung,fava, navy,adzuki, or some other kind are not difficult to add to soups, mixed greens, stews, lasagna, or dishes; you might crush them with spices and flavors as a plunge for vegetables. Indeed, even canned, however as long as they're low in sodium and washed (this eliminates 40 to 50 percent of the sodium), they're not difficult to eat, reasonable, and wealthy in sustenance.

8. Spices and flavourings:
Spices and flavors make nutritious fixings (counting vegetables, fish, and plant-based protein sources) taste better — in addition, they assist us with bringing down our salt and added sugar consumption, which we want to restrict and add to solid maturing and diminished irritation.
Significant revelations are arising on the phytochemical, mitigating, and other unique characteristics of spices and flavors themselves, as well. They're additionally one more key component of the Mediterranean eating regimen, which has the nearest relationship with living long and living great.

A couple of our top picks? Ginger and garlic, basil, chives (famous for its calming and hostile to sickness benefits), rosemary, cinnamon, turmeric,nutmeg, cumin, (solid mitigating characteristics), and red pepper.